I0440380

*Maintaining Your Weight: Staying in the Center*

By Doris Richardson-Edsell

Copyright April 2014 by Doris Richardson-Edsell

# Table of Contents

## Healthy Beginnings: Helping People to Stay Well

I know people may not want to hear about cleaning up their diet, but I have found that it really has helped me. I enjoy foods that I never thought I would, such as eggplant and spinach. I love spinach!

It seems like it takes a long time to lose weight because you have to change so much. You have to focus on health-instead of cheating on your diet! You are only cheating yourself!

It has been a wonderful 5 years because I feel so much better and an added effect of cleaning up my diet has been a weight loss. The weight loss also happened because I began exercising more frequently. I jog, ride a bike and teach yoga.

### Bucket lists

Today, my goal is to help others to develop lifestyle changes that can lead to health and wellness in mind, body and spirit.
This is my *bucket list!*
To be the person who helps others to grow stronger and feel better.
Remember that lifestyle changes may be difficult to attain. It may take some time to be where you want to be but it is worth the struggle.

When you make the changes that you need to make, you will be stronger and feel better.
You will have more energy and your state of mind will be more balanced. Treat your body well, and your body will thank you! Eat nutritious foods and exercise every day of your life.

It does not have to be strenuous exercise, but you should do something active every single day of your life. Do not make excuses for not getting out there to take your daily walk. Find "like minded" people who are trying their best to stay healthy. They can help you to stay on your road to wellness.

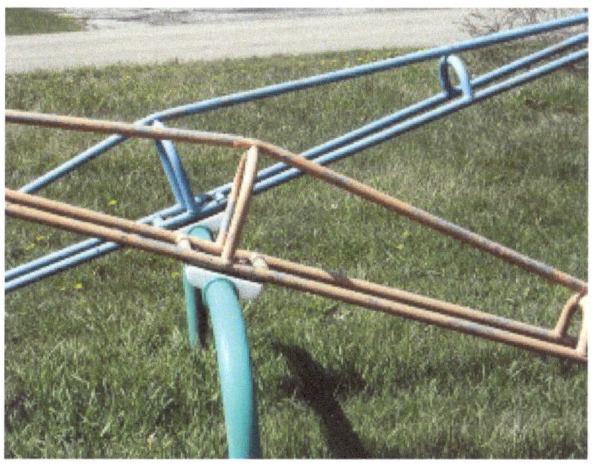

*Think of your life as a teeter-totter- you swing up and down with your weight. Make today the beginning of not only losing weight, but believing that you can also keep it off. Find friends who also struggle with their weight, and band together to build strength.*

## Maintaining Your Weight: Staying in the Center

### *Where is your center?*

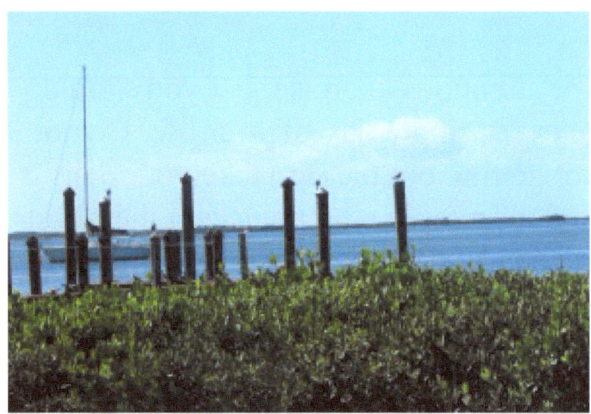

### *Birds together finding ways to their center*

My center is clear, and I have a friend, Christine who would agree. She believes in this theory on maintaining your weight where your center is your bliss!

### *To the right are your good choices*

To the right are the foods and exercises that you need to do. To the left are the sweet indulgences that you may want all the time.

And staying in the center with some tiny bits of sweetness is a good goal.

### *Remember there are many other things to do besides thinking about your life in the sweet lane*

Exercise is a great distraction for those hungry days, and if you crave too many sweets it is probably a good idea to put more protein in your diet.

More grains such as quinoa, millet or barley can help you feel full because they are full of protein and fiber. Begin to learn how to cook grains; like the grain rice, the others cook the same way; equal parts of water and grains.

And the fiber in the grains keeps you full, so having a lot of fibrous foods is what to do to keep those hungry times away. Other powerful fibrous foods are veggies and fruits. When you are hungry between meals, have a healthy vegetable or fruit snack.

### *The Center Can Bring You Harmony*

Make today your first day toward a healthier you. Go shopping and pick up some healthy grains. Try different ones; amaranth and even legumes such as split peas and lentils are packed with protein.

If you begin to eat healthier foods, you will begin to crave the sweets less and less; bringing you into your center where you feel balanced and healthy.

## What is in your Future? Do you have some goals?

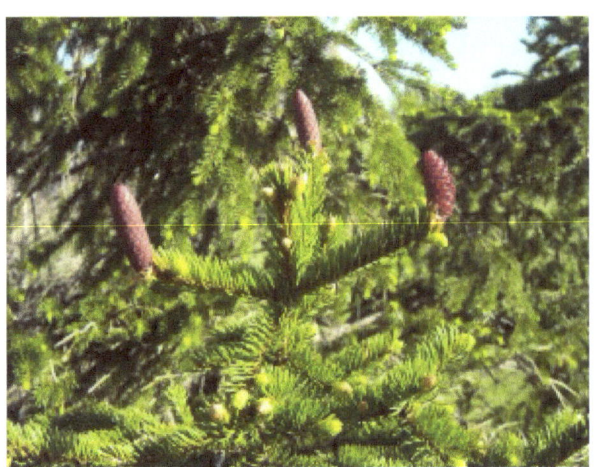

*When I see all the budding on the trees I begin to think that it is time for me to make some changes too!*

Everything these days seems to move toward what your goals are, and how to attain them. In college I learned an old saying about goals: ***Choose, Get, Keep.*** You first choose a realistic goal, write it down, and when you get the goal attained, you find ways to keep it; and that is the hardest part; being able to keep your hard earned goal for the rest of your life.

We have goals for career, money, health and wellness.

In order to plant the seed of losing and keeping weight at bay, you must realize that it is a fragile skill when it comes to not only taking it off but maintaining it for the rest of your life. That is the real deal!

Because of this long term goal plan, you must begin to think about your planning in a sense of a lifelong commitment, therefore, a healthy living goal or lifestyle change that is long lasting. That is why diets don't work. And the word diet has the word "die" right in it! That says it all!

### *Your plan? Three simple steps*

1. **Portion Control.** This one is so very important. You need to measure everything. Only have a half cup of grains and pasta. And remember that a piece of meat is the size of a deck of cards. If you want some cheese, it is the size of a few dominos!

Portion control is the main reason that most people's lifestyle change does not work. We think we are only eating one portion, but we just ate four.

2. **Daily exercise. Don't go with the 3 days a week routine.** If you exercise by doing something every single day of your life, you will not have to remember when you did it last; and find something that you like so that you keep on doing it.

3. **Limit Eating Out:** Eat most of your meals at home so that you know exactly what you are eating and how much.

I only eat out once a week. It is special, and I always remember that they are going to give me at least 2 portions, sometimes more, so I ask for a doggy bag early, before I get to thinking about just one more bite!

***How do you change the not so good habits into good ones?***

***How can you change yourself?***

You have to start thinking about your plan of action; especially related to sticking to the program. You have to stay on the plan for at least 3 months to have any bad habits disappear to be replaced with good habits such as taking a daily walk, or loving baby carrots.

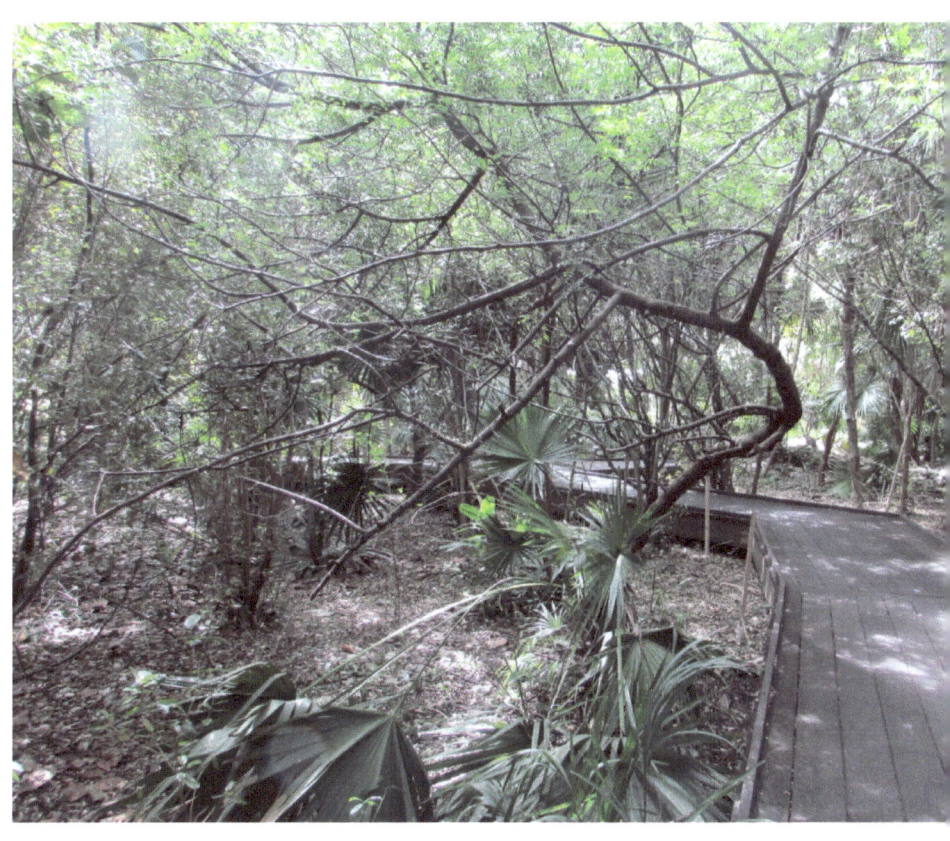

**Take a walk every single day of your life**

## What are you eating? Some Functional Foods

*There are many foods which are packed with vitamins and minerals to help you stay healthy and well. Did you know that they are called Functional Foods?*

The first Functional Food that I think about are the orange ones! Carotenoids- they are the B-Carotene in carrots, orange fruits, butternut squash and cantaloupe. Great for your health and wellness; the yellower the better!

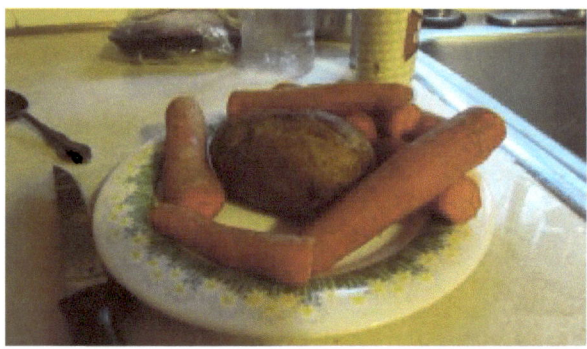

*Back to basics; steamed carrots and potatoes*

Here are a few more functional foods:

**Lycopene** is found in foods such as tomato products.

**Lutein** is found in dark green veggies such as kale, spinach, collard greens, eggs, corn and citrus.

Onions, garlic, scallions, leeks and chives are called- Diallyl Sulfides and the name for strawberries, raspberries, pomegranates, and berries and walnuts are called- Ellagic Acids

*OMEGA 3's* you have all heard of the Omega – 3 s and how important they are. You do not have to take these fatty acids in pill form if you eat them. The fatty acid- a-linolenic acid is found in flax seeds, flax oil, walnuts, canola oil, soybean oil, sardines in oil and Atlantic salmon.

For some Eicosapentaenoic Acid- you can eat some herring, salmon, Wild Alaskan Salmon, blue fin tuna.

And finally, you can find Docosahexaenoic Acid in Atlantic salmon, Blue Fin Tuna, Mackerel and Omega-3 enriched eggs. And if it sounds complicated, it really is not. Here are some tips on how to get your pre and probiotics.

**PREBIOTIC-** Whole grains, especially oatmeal, flax and barley, greens, berries, bananas, legumes, onions, garlic, honey and leeks.

**PROBIOTIC-** This is your yogurt. But it does not have to be only dairy yogurt. You can find probiotics in soy, almond or coconut yogurt, and fermented dairy and non-dairy products such as sauerkraut and fermented soy such as miso and tempeh.

**Other functional Foods:**

**Phenols-** they are in apples, pears, citrus fruit, parsley, carrots, broccoli, cabbage, cucumbers, squash, yams and tomatoes.

**Lignan's-** they are found in flax seed, rye

**Flavonoids-** found in berries, especially the dark berries, cherries, red grapes and tea– especially green tea.

### *Your diet and what you should be eating*

When you are choosing what to eat, you want to stick to the basics such as discovering the resources that are available to you such as Getting Started with *My Plate*. It replaced the food pyramid a few years ago, making it easier to understand what you should be eating. This government program is online for your convenience- ChooseMyPlate.gov

### The recommendations on healthy eating include:

Enjoy your food but eat less

Avoid oversized portions

Make half of your plate fruits and veggies!

Switch to fat free or low fat milk (1%)

Make at least half of your grains– whole grains

Look at the sodium in foods- especially products such as soups, breads and frozen meals, and choose foods with low sodium numbers.

Drink water instead of sugary drinks

Recommendations on Healthy Eating in part from the US government resource: MyPlate.gov. Fall/Winter 2011

# Do you want healthy digestion? Focus on good food combinations

*A Healthy diet and Exercise can deliver you great health*

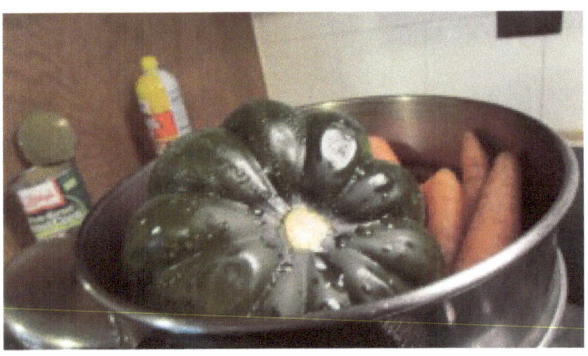

Some steamed veggies

Today there are many new diet and exercise tips but good nutrition tips have been around for many years. Author Howard Hay developed The Hay Diet in 1939 and his theories are still very sound advice today.

The theory is on the importance of food combinations for healthy digestion.

Dr. Hay pointed out that a combination of high-protein and high-starch foods has appalling effects on the digestive system. Dr. Hay himself was troubled by painful digestion for many years related to chronic inflammation of his kidneys, high blood pressure and a badly dilated heart. When he changed his eating habits, his symptoms disappeared.

*Here is Dr. Hay's General Theory on Food: The Hay Diet*

1. Carbohydrates should never be eaten in combination with proteins and acidic foods

2. Vegetables, salads and fruits should make up the bulk of the diet

3. Proteins, carbohydrates and fats should be eaten only in small amounts. Only wholegrain, unrefined carbohydrates should be used.

4. Refined and processed foods should be avoided

5. There should be an interval of at least 4 hours between meals of different types of foods

6. One meal a day should be based on starchy foods, another on protein foods and the third should be alkaline foods. (Some alkaline foods have a neutral pH such as tap water, most spring water. A pH of 8 foods- apples almonds, grapefruit, corn, mushrooms, turnip, soy, bell pepper, radish, pineapple, cherries, wild rice, apricot, strawberries, bananas. pH 9- avocado, green tea, lettuce, celery, peas, sweet potatoes, eggplant, green beans, beets, blueberries, pears, grapes, Kiwi, tangerines, figs, dates, mangoes, papaya pH 10- spinach, broccoli, artichoke, brussel sprouts, cabbage, cauliflower, carrots, cucumber, lemon, limes, seaweed, asparagus, radish, collard greens, onions.)

*ACIDIC FOODS THAT CAUSE DIGESTIVE ISSUES–*
*carbonated water, club soda, energy drinks- pH3*

**pH 4** Popcorn, cream cheese, buttermilk, prunes, pastries, cheese, pork, beer, wine, black tea, pickles, chocolate, roasted nuts, vinegar, sweet and low, equal, nutra sweet.

**pH 5** Purified water, distilled water, coffee, sweetened fruit juice, pistachios, beef, white bread, peanuts, nuts, wheat

**pH 6-** Most grains, eggs, fish, tea, cooked beans, cooked spinach, soy milk, coconut, lima beans, plums, brown rice, barley, cocoa, oats, liver, oyster, salmon.

What is really causing your indigestion or bloating?

Indigestion is caused by too much acid in the stomach. What to avoid: Alcohol, strong tea, coffee, fizzy drinks, meat extracts, acidic foods such as pickles and vinegar, hot spicy foods, unripe fruit, cheese.

*Discomfort or bloating?*

Other common triggers of digestive issues are stress, eating too fast/hurried, insufficient chewing, long gaps between meals which leads to binge eating; swallowing air, and bloating. Tobacco use also triggers gastric acid secretion.

## The basic principles of the Hay Diet:

1. Understand that starch begins to ferment in the stomach as soon as the salivary enzyme ptyalin is destroyed by gastric juices.

2. Healthy foods in the right combinations can greatly improve digestion

3. All foods comprise of one of the 5 nutrients and it is vital to identify the dominant nutrient in a meal, and proportion accordingly:

## THE 5 NUTRIENT GROUPS

**Starches**- bread, pasta rice

**Proteins**- meat, fish, eggs cheese, soy

**Sugars**- firm fruit such as fresh banana, honey, sweet preserves

**Acids**- soft fruits such as peaches, plums

**Fats**- oil, mayonnaise, egg yolk

Carbohydrates fall into 2 groups- the sugars and starches.

*Example: Remember that proteins, carbs and fats should be eaten in small amounts. Veggies, salads and fruits make up the bulk of your diet with 4 hours between meals.*

**Breakfast** (starch)

Oatmeal with almond milk (carbs)

Sliced banana and pineapple

**Lunch (based on protein)**

Soy burger (9 grams protein), slice wholegrain bread, lettuce salad with raw veggies such as cucumbers, carrots

**Dinner (alkaline food focused)**

Veggie mix of broccoli, red bell peppers, and 1/2 cup brown rice (limited portion of rice- a healthy carb). Fruit cup of mangoes and papaya (a bit acidic due to their soft nature.)

Snack- apple- hard fruit the best for low acidity

**Exercise**

Do not forget about exercise in your healthy living plan. Exercise such as a fast walk in the morning helps the digestion of foods in the body.

Tips on some food combos and indigestion from the book by: Dries, J. & Dries, I (2002) *The Food Combining Bible.* Hammersmith, London. Harper-Collins.

## What to do with Kale? Mix With Beans and Grains

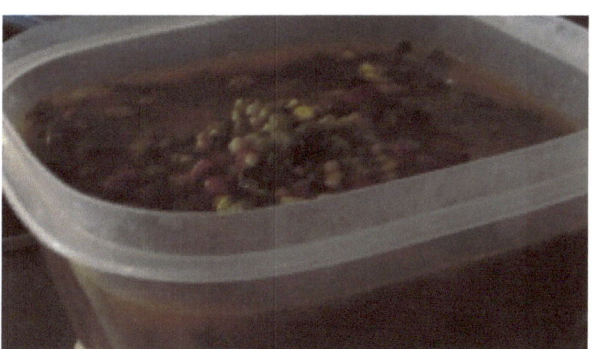

*The beauty of making soup is that it can help you with increasing the fiber in your diet*

Did you know that there are many studies on the fact that people who eat soup are thinner?

Why not give soup a try.

### Veggie Soup with Split peas and beans

Some recipes that are good and packed with protein include adding grains, legumes and beans.
Here is a recipe for a great veggie soup with kidney beans, split peas and kale.

For many people who are sodium restricted, making your own soup is a very good idea because you alone control the amount of salt you put in. And there are many different kinds of spices that you can use in a recipe that perk up the flavor without adding any salt.

For most of my soup recipes, I start out in a separate frying pan sprinkled with 2 teaspoons of olive oil, adding teaspoon of very finely chopped ginger, a clove of chopped garlic, and 1 small chopped white onion. I simmer for about 5 minutes and put to the side to add to my soup.

### Starting the Soup

I always start out with 2 cups of tomato or V-8 juice, adding 2 cups of water or veggie broth. Remember to use the low sodium kind, especially if you are on a sodium restricted diet.

I add the onion, garlic and ginger and then I begin to add 1/2 cup raw soy beans, 1/2 cup quinoa, 1/2 cup  split peas (they need to be rinsed thoroughly for stones/bugs) first because they take about 1/2 hour to cook. After the grains, legumes and soy beans are almost done, I begin to add my other veggies such as 2 cups fresh kale, 1 cup frozen corn, 1 can of kidney beans, rinsed well.

Simmer for another 30 minutes or longer depending on how you like your veggies.

Each cup of this soup is packed with fiber and protein.

## *Kale Chips*

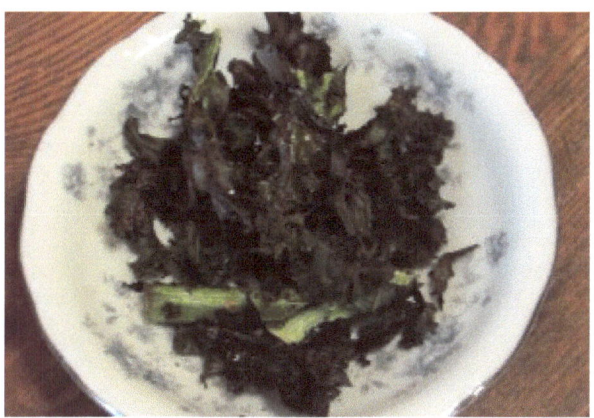

## Crunchy like potato chips!

For an added appetizer, I also roast some kale in a pre-heated 350 degree oven.

Use parchment paper lined on a cookie sheet. Add washed and dry pieces of kale to the cookie sheet, (you can cut off the stems if you want smaller pieces) sprinkle with garlic powder and drizzle with 1 tablespoon olive oil and cook in an over 350 degrees for about 10 minutes until the edges are brown.

Eat right away as a snack or as an appetizer for your soup.

## Perfect Timing

*Believing in yourself and your dreams*

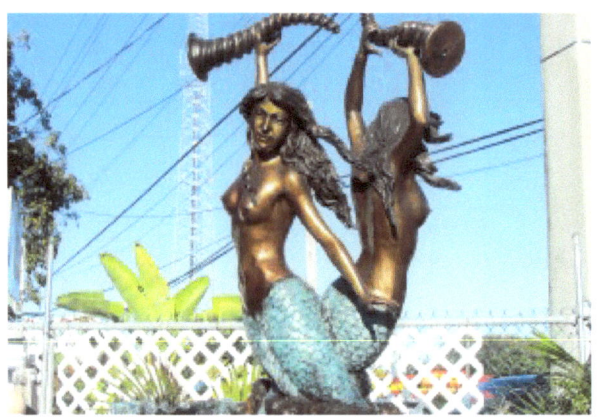

*They are in our imagination and dreams, helping others to see clearly*

Is there a perfect time to do anything?

Or do you purposefully put off things until the right time? I believe that you may have to work on a *step-by-step* way toward any goals that you may be putting off until tomorrow.

### In Your Dreams
So many people live with dreams in their hearts that are not accomplished because they are waiting for the perfect time.
Forget about perfection and begin to plunge along into the items on your list of things you are passionate about.

### Completing your Education
If it is finishing your education, take just one course on a

topic you are truly interested in, and with that momentum you will move toward the next class, getting closer to your goal.

### *Weight Reduction and Maintenance: One of the most difficult accomplishments for many people*

If it is about your weight, and I know that this is a difficult goal, but take some baby steps toward where you want to be. Start eliminating those triggers foods that you have around in the house that ruin your efforts at a healthy day. This one step can get you on the road toward wellness. Be a conscious shopper. Do not go to the grocery store hungry. Do not buy foods that you know you have no control over such as even one donut!

### *Exercise Helps with Your Mind, Body and Soul*
Be an avid exerciser. Do not say you will wait until it is warmer outside. Do go out there, and bundle up.
Do not say you will do some exercise 3 days a week. Do something every day.

Exercise can be your distraction from food. Exercise can also lift your mood. Exercise is one of the most important aspects of your goal toward wellness and continual health throughout your life.

Get out there and stop procrastinating — there really is no perfect time to begin, so begin now.

## In the Groove of Weight Loss and Maintenance

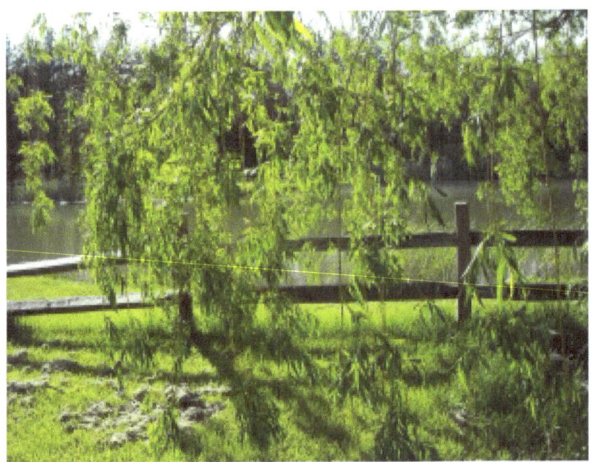

*Looking at green is so good. The weeping willow hovers, swaying in the breeze*

***What is it that you need to do in order to keep up the momentum of weight loss and maintenance?***
I find that I fall off the wagon at times, and then need to jump back on by making my list of the things that I may have forgotten about.

Whether you are a beginner, or a maintainer of weight, it can catch up with you! If you do not continue to "watch those calories," they will show up on your thighs!

***Some tips on Weight Loss and Maintenance***
1. **Eating slowly:** When you eat mindfully, you are concentrating on your food, and taste of each bite.

You always sit down, never eating on the run, or standing, or in your car!

2. **Watch your portions:** When I slip up on my maintenance goal, it is usually about how much I am eating- not what I am eating. I tend to eat wholesome, whole foods, but at times I have to get the measuring cup out, and my theory? Never eat more than 1/2 cup of anything. And when you measure out that cup of pasta, even if you move up to the full cup, it is not a lot of pasta! That is why I try my best to fill up on some good foods such as veggies, especially the green ones such as spinach and fennel.

3. **Exercise Daily:** If you try to do something 3 days a week, before you know it you did it yesterday!! Oh yeah, I forgot, I did not do it yesterday, did I?

My theory is to do something every day of the week and then you will not procrastinate. And if you exercise every day, you do not have to work as hard every day. You can still step it up a bit a few days a week. For example, I may just walk on Mondays and Tuesdays, but on Wednesdays I run, on Thursdays I do yoga; on Fridays I ride my bike. There is evidence that "changing it up" is a good idea. You cannot do the same thing day after day and expect different results. So be creative.

4. **Enlist others in your quest toward wellness and health:** There must be someone who needs to lose weight that you know. They can become your cardio buddy who reminds you that it is time to exercise.

The more the merrier! Form a group where you get together and talk about how everyone is doing in their weight loss and maintenance efforts.

## Where did I leave my happy thoughts?

### *Moving on to the positive side of living*

Like the *Peter Pan* story, all that you need is to think a happy thought and things get better in life. And there is research on the theory that people who smile more, stay more positive and are optimistic, not only live longer, they are happier people.

When you want to changes something about yourself and you feel a lot of negative energy inside how do you move that negative energy out of your system?

Water scenes always work for me! I am just floating aimlessly down the *Inlet of Life. I let it all go* and think about my own breath of life, meditating on the clouds and singing a beautiful song in my head that never stops. That is my positive mantra.

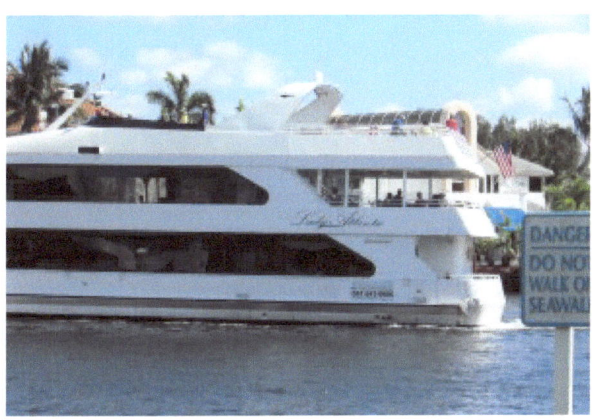

*You can take a trip down your ocean of life, slowly ridding yourself from negativity and then you will feel so much better*

You can work on yourself in a positive way if you begin to realize that you may be standing in your own way of the *happy thoughts* that you are wishing for.

If you are like me, and you dwell too much on past things that happened to you, you have to stop it. It may be easier said than done, but you have to start somewhere to protect yourself from yourself.
People who look at you from the outside may not even notice that you have difficulties and you may be able to cover it up quite effectively but you cannot cover it up from yourself.

Even if you have had more loss than most people, you need to take life *by the horns* and find pleasant ways to come back to the you that you know so well; that *Peter Pan like* person who does not need to act grown up all the time.

Take some time to watch *Peter Pan* just one more time. Robin Williams in *Hook* creates that perfect person who has grown up only to realize that he was a much better person in mind, body and spirit when he believed that he would never grow up– and that he could stop time, and stay in that child-like moment with just a happy thought!

### *My Peter Pan Ways: You are what you believe you are*

And always remember that you are what you think you are. If you feel fat, you are fat, and if you feel thin and beautiful, that is what you are. If you know you cannot lose weight, you will never do it, but if you believe it is possible, your weight loss goal is within your reach.

## Loving What Your Eat and Eating What You Love

### *Organization is the key to a great healthy living plan*

Have a clean kitchen where it is a pleasure to make meals; your counters are clean, and you have enough food in you fridge to create great, low calorie meals with plenty of fruits and vegetables.

### *More of the good Carbs Please!*

What are the good carbs? They are the ones that take a long time to get through your body; rice, grains, fruits and vegetables. They are the color in your meals; the bright red bell peppers, the fresh orange carrots and the greener than green collard greens! You can eat them raw, you can eat them blanched, and you can eat them in soups. And veggies should be your main staple because you can eat as much as you want!

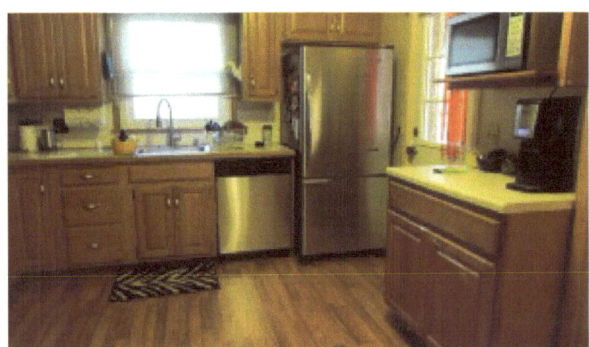

*Organize your kitchen so that everything is where it needs to be. Make it a clean environment where you can make a nice meal*

When I think of eating, I think of fresh fruits and veggies. I love to eat a variety of foods that are colorful and tasty. Crispy veggies with some brown rice are a great meal. If you begin to enjoy the low fat- complex carbohydrates instead of the fatty foods, you really begin to enjoy what you are eating.

### Taking control

Begin to take control of your eating by only eating when you are hungry. Many people go by the clock with eating. Allow your body to tell you when it needs care.

### Activity

When you are active every day of your life, you learn the cues of your body's hunger. You become hungry because you are moving and grooving!

### Realism

If you are trying to lose some weight, stop punishing yourself with unrealistic goals of losing a lot of weight. Make mini goals of losing 3 pounds, not 20. The pounds will come off if you stick to it.

### Your body size

Stop it! Stop looking at yourself and thinking that you look terrible. You need to begin cherishing the way you look even if you are not where you want to be. Striving for perfection is not the key to long lasting weight control. And looking at the commercials on TV telling you that you can be a 10 may be very unrealistic. Do not send yourself critical messages about your body; love your body.

## *Be Mindful*

Always be mindful of eating. Do not sit in front of the TV eating because this one thing will sabotage all your efforts for your day.

Eat slowly and mindfully, small bits of food cut up, whatever you need to do to slow you down. Look at your food, use colorful, small plates that exaggerate how much you are eating, and of course- chew your food well.

## Appendix:

## Minerals in Nutrition

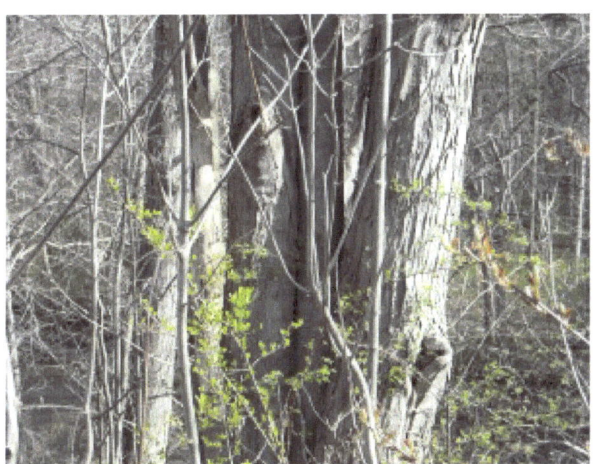

## MINERALS

To help people understand nutrition better, I am devoting a post on essential minerals that the body needs. There are 2 classes of micronutrients, vitamins and minerals. Vitamins are complex and organic, serving primarily as coenzymes or regulators of body metabolism.

Minerals are simple elements with important roles in both structure and function of the body.

## ORGANICS

**Eating organically grown foods is important because if the soil is deficient in minerals, the food grown in that soil can be deficient.**

**What are the major minerals?**

**There are 7 major minerals:** Calcium, Phosphorus, Sodium, Potassium, Magnesium, Chloride, and Sulfur.

**The trace elements are:** Iron, Iodine, Zinc, Manganese, Copper, Chromium, Cobalt, Molybdenum and Fluoride.

Our body requires a plentiful supply of organic minerals. Our soil, filled with microbes, breaks down the inorganic minerals and the plants absorb them. This process renders the minerals organic and able to be assimilated into the body.

1. **Calcium** is the skeletal mineral, needed for growth and development, keeping the heart healthy, and for muscle activity. Calcium is the mineral that is present in the largest amount in the body. Calcium aides in the formation of bones and teeth, helping in metabolic functions such as blood clotting, nerve transmission, muscle contraction and relaxation. Good sources include milk, yogurt, cheese, orange juice, spinach, white beans, tofu and bread.

You need the proper intake of Vitamin D, or bone development can be impeded. With the loss of bone, osteoporosis can form.

2. **Phosphorus** is associated with calcium in the body. Most phosphorus is found in the skeleton and teeth, with calcium. Phosphorus works with proteins, lipids, and carbohydrates to produce energy, build and repair tissue and help maintain a good pH level. Good sources: milk and lean meat

3. **Sodium-** about 95% of sodium is found in extracellular fluid as free ionized sodium. This sodium guards the body

water outside of the cells, regulating acid-base balance in the body. Sodium helps to maintain muscle action. High sodium can lead to high blood pressure. Spinach and celery are fairly high in sodium.

4. **Potassium** found inside cells where it guards intercellular water. Some is found in extracellular fluid which is good for muscle activity. Potassium inside helps balance sodium outside of cells to maintain osmotic pressure. Taking too much potassium can lead to hyperkalemia and cardiac arrhythmias. Good sources: legumes, whole grains, fruits, leafy green veggies, broccoli, potatoes, meat and milk.

5. **Magnesium** is found in all body cells aiding in good bone, muscle, and tissue health. Good sources include: whole grains, nuts, soybeans, cocoa, seafood, dried beans, peas and green veggies.

6. **Chloride** is found in extracellular fluid to help control water balance and acid-base balance. Some ionized chloride is found in gastrointestinal secretions. When a loss of gastric fluids occurs with vomiting and diarrhea it can cause chloride deficiency with muscle cramps and disturbed acid-base balance.

7. **Sulfur** is in all body cells. It aides in protein structure, enzyme activity and detoxification reactions. Sulfur can be found in meat, eggs, milk, cheese, legumes and nuts.

**The trace elements (there are 9)**

**Iron:** Found in abundance in nature, it is essential to life. The main function is to combine with protein and copper in making hemoglobin. Iron promotes the metabolism of protein. Sources: liver, oyster, heart, lean meat, green leafy veggies, brewer's yeast, molasses, prunes, apricots, peaches, bananas, eggs, whole grains, pumpkin, sunflower, sesame seeds, kelp, parsley, soybeans, lentils, and almonds.

**Iodine** is "the energy mineral" needed for the health of the thyroid gland, and the production of thyroxin, the hormone produced by the thyroid. Most food sources have little iodine. Though some plants grown in iodine-rich soil and seafood have higher concentrations.

Found in Kelp, seafood, fish liver oils, garlic, watercress, pineapple, egg yolks, turnip greens, mustard greens, watermelon, cucumber, asparagus and green pepper.

**Zinc** is important for the absorption of B vitamins and linoleic acid, an essential fatty acid that helps keep the skin healthy. Zinc is helpful in speeding up the healing process. Zinc is one of the most important mineral for the immune system as it assists antibodies, white blood cells, the thymus gland, and hormone function. Pregnant women need to take adequate zinc to assist in normal fetal growth and development. Oral contraceptives can destroy zinc. Soy protein, glucose, lactose and red wine enhance zinc absorption. Animal and fish sources are more readily absorbed as they contain amino acids that bind with zinc.

**Manganese** is one of the essential trace elements needed for metabolism of carbohydrates, fats and proteins. It is the "Love" mineral because animals will not suckle their young if deficient in manganese. It is important for healthy nerves, normal reproduction, and the production of breast milk. Sources: seeds, nuts, fresh wheat germ, legumes, buckwheat, green leafy veggies, oranges, grapefruit, apricots, peas, kelp, egg yolk, dried fruit.

**Copper** is absorbed in the small intestines and stored in many tissues. Excessive Copper storage in the body can lead to Wilson's disease. Found in meat, liver, seafood, whole grains, legumes, nuts.

**Chromium** is absorbed in association with Zinc and excreted in the kidneys. Chromium is associated with glucose metabolism, potentiating the action of insulin. Found in whole grains and cereals, Brewer's yeast, animal protein food.

**Cobalt** is absorbed as a component of vitamin B12, and stored in the liver. Cobalt functions with vitamin B12. A deficiency exists only if deficient also in vitamin B12. Cobalt is found only in animal foods that contain vitamin B12, therefore, vegetarians; especially vegans who consume no dairy are at risk of deficiency unless they take a supplement.

**Molybdenum** is readily absorbed and excreted by the kidneys. Found in legumes, whole grains, milk, organ meat, fish and fish products, leafy vegetables.

**Fluoride** absorbed by the small intestine and excreted by the kidneys. Fluoride accumulates in bones and teeth, which increases hardness. Found in fish, tea, drinking water, foods cooked in fluorinated water.

Taken in part from: Schlenker, E. and Long, S. (2007). *Williams' Essentials of Nutrition and Diet Therapy.* St Louis, Mo. Mosby, Inc.

Mahan, K. and Escott-Stump, S. (2008). *Krause's Food and Nutrition Therapy.* St. Louis, Mo. Saunders.

## Vitamins are important for our overall health: Our brain food

It is well established and researched that vitamins need to be in our diets, hopefully through what we eat or supplemented daily. B vitamins have been of special note due to their ability to help with many things such as memory, neurological functioning and other brain abilities such as concentration.

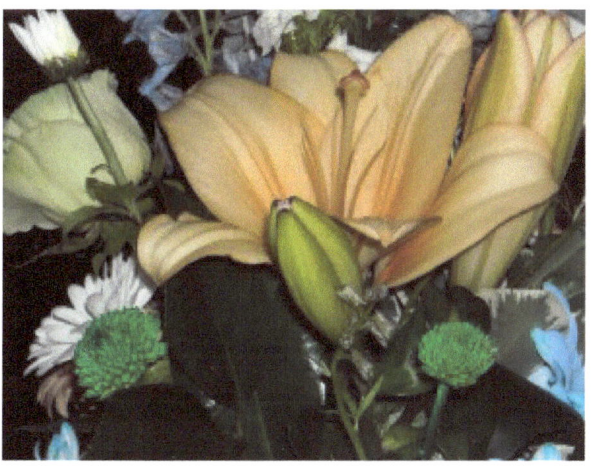

The following are some tips on the importance of vitamins. As you read, you will see that many of the water soluble help with overall mental functioning and are needed for sleep problems such as insomnia, memory and concentration.

There are symptoms of deficiency and toxicity in vitamins and many people do not know that there are maximum dosages. In an article on natural nutritional supplements I came across this good overview of vitamins.

## VITAMIN A

Deficiency: frequent colds, respiratory problems

Toxicity: Aches and pains, poor appetite, yellowing of the skin, weight loss, sore eyes, enlarged liver, decalcification of bones

Found in: Green leafy veggies, liver, eggs, whole milk, cream, carrots, fruits, cod liver oil

Recommended daily allowance for adults: 6,000IU/ 3000 IU children

## VITAMIN B1 (Thiamine)

Deficiency: mental confusion, depression, fatigue, apathy, anxiety, inability to concentrate, sensitivity to noise, low blood pressure

Toxicity: Water soluble so excess is not stored in the body

Found in: Dairy products, brewer's yeast, bran, mushrooms, dark green vegetables, organ meats

Recommended daily allowance for adults: 1 mg-1.5mg

## B2 (Riboflavin)

Deficiency:  Red tongue, cracks in the corners of the mouth, dizzy, watery or bloodshot eyes, hair loss, brain and nervous system changes, mental sluggishness, depression

Toxicity: Water soluble

Found in: Dairy products, organ meat, brewer's yeast, poultry, fish, eggs dried beans, peanuts

Recommended daily allowance for adults: 10mg

## B2 (Niacin)

Deficiency: Depression, insomnia, weakness, mental confusion, red-tipped tongue, sore mouth, dermatitis, excessive gas, irritability

Toxicity: Water soluble

Found in Lean meats, peanuts, brewer's yeast, wheat germ, liver, fish poultry

Recommended daily allowance for adults: 18 mg (men) 13 mg (women)

## B5 (Pantothenic Acid)

Deficiency: Fatigue, sleep disturbances, depression, constipation, low blood pressure, irritability, burning feet

Toxicity: Water Soluble

Found in: Organ meats, bran, peanuts, brewer's yeast

Recommended daily allowance for adults: 10mg

## B6 (Pyridoxine)

Deficiency: Mental confusion, irritability, depression, anxiety, numbness or cramps in the hands and feet, insomnia, nausea in the morning, anemia, water retention, PMS symptoms

Toxicity: Water soluble

Found in: Meat fish, peanuts, soybeans, bananas, whole grains, spinach, broccoli, legumes

Recommended allowance for adults: 2.3 mg

## B12 (Coalmine)

Deficiency: Pernicious anemia, numbness, neurological changes, poor reflexes, apathy, poor concentration, confusion, poor memory

Toxicity: Water Soluble

Found in: Eggs, meat, poultry, fish, dairy, brewer's yeast

Recommended Daily Allowance for Adults: 6mcg

## Folic Acid

Deficiency: Anemia, poor digestion, constipation, deterioration of nervous system, apathy, withdrawn, irritability, poor memory

Toxicity: Can mask B12 pernicious anemia, water soluble

Found in: Green leafy veggies, wheat germ, dried beans, and peas

Recommended daily allowances for adults: 100mcg

### Choline

Deficiency: Low levels prevent adequate conversion to memory neurotransmitters (acetylcholine)

Recommended daily allowances: none established

Found in Lecithin, egg yolks

(There have been recommendations on treatment of memory- 10g daily)

### Inositol

Deficiency: Poor sleep, anxiety, panic attacks, depression

Toxicity: unknown

Recommended daily allowances for adults: none established

Found in: whole grains, lecithin, liver, brewer's yeast

### Biotin

Deficiency: Fatigue, depression, skin disorders, muscle pain

Toxicity: unknown

Found in: yeast, pork and lamb liver, egg yolks, nuts - especially peanuts

Recommended daily allowance: none established however our own bodies make about 300mg daily

## *Vitamin C*

Deficiency: Fatigue, loss of appetite, sore gums, slow wound healing, aching joints, bruising easily, frequent infections

Toxicity: rare, water soluble

Recommended daily allowances for adults: 20mg

Found in: citrus fruits, cauliflower, Brussels sprouts, broccoli

## **Vitamin D**

Deficiency: Rickets, rheumatoid pain, exhaustion, hypothyroidism

Toxicity: Calcium storage and calcification in the soft tissues of the body, frequent thirst and urination, nausea and vomiting, weakness and loss of appetite

Found in: Cod liver oil, sunlight, egg yolk, fish, added to dairy products

Recommended daily allowance in adults: 400IU

## *Vitamin E*

Deficiency: Restless, fatigue, insomnia, menopausal symptoms, muscle wasting and liver damage

Toxicity: High Blood pressure may occur if high doses are taken at onset of use

Found in: Wheat germ, cold pressed oils such as sunflower, safflower, spinach, sweet potatoes, almonds, walnuts, broccoli

Recommended daily allowance for adults: 15 IU

## Vitamin K

Deficiency: Bleeding disorders, hemorrhaging

Toxicity: Natural K is not toxic

Found in: leafy green veggies, tomatoes, pork, liver and carrots

Recommended daily allowance: none established

(500 mcg: antibiotics and sulfa drugs can destroy Vitamin K which contains intestinal bacteria. Acidophilus cultures 3 times daily can help replace the friendly flora)

Taken in part from: *Natural Nutrition Supplements*. Joan Mathews Larson at http://www.joanmathews larson.com/HRC_2006/Depression

www.ingramcontent.com/pod-product-compliance
Lightning Source LLC
Chambersburg PA
CBHW051128290526
45796CB00001B/4